SPECIA
squa
healthy col

What Your Poo Says About You

Dr. Alison Chen, ND

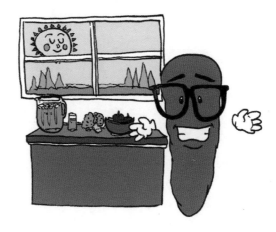

ILLUSTRATED BY JEREMY WAT

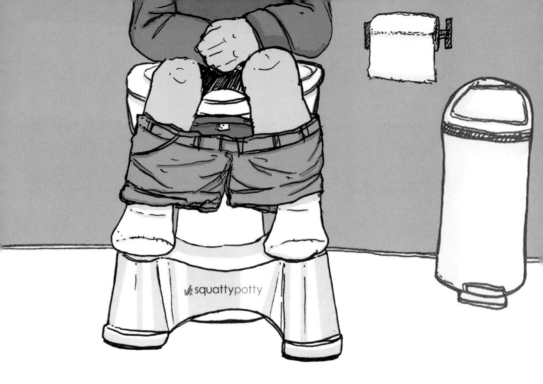

Your poo not only tells you
all about your digestion,
But also your immune system,
stress levels and nutrition.

Healthy bowel movements
should occur 1-3 times per day,
Every time you eat a meal
signals your GI to work and play.

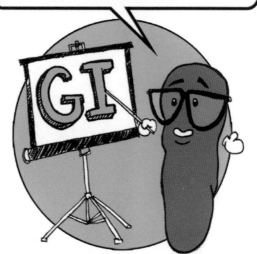

GI STANDS FOR GASTROINTESTINAL TRACT.

Cannonball

Those little lumps are stubborn
 and often hard to please.
Remember to drink lots of water
 and relax to feel at ease.

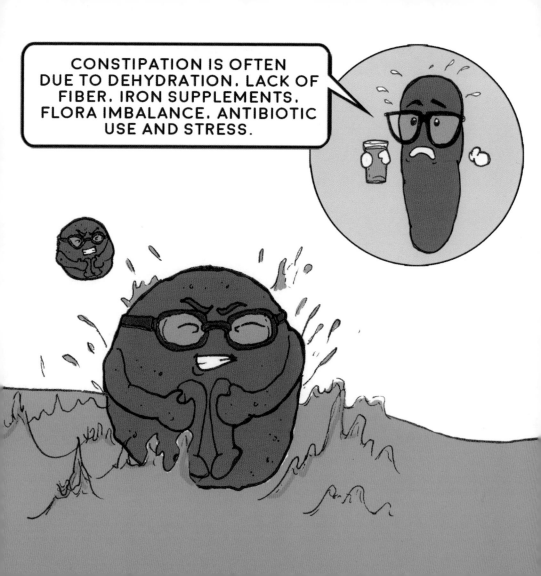

Torpedo Bum

This high-pressured turd
  is painful to pass,
Without greens and hydration
  he'll make a big splash.

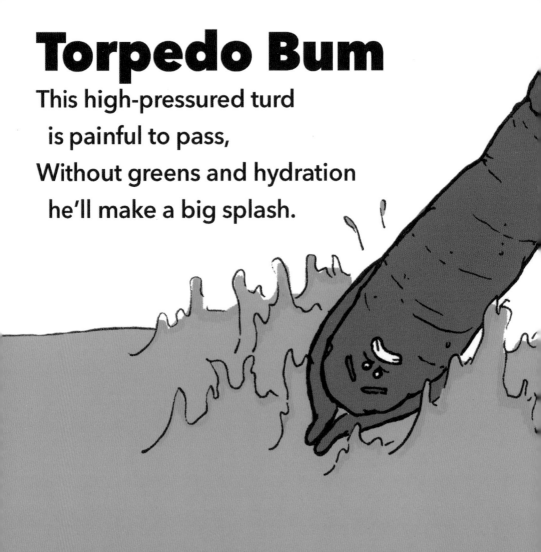

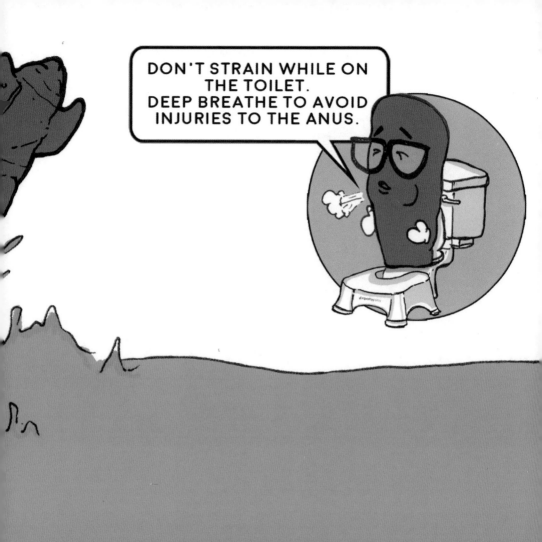

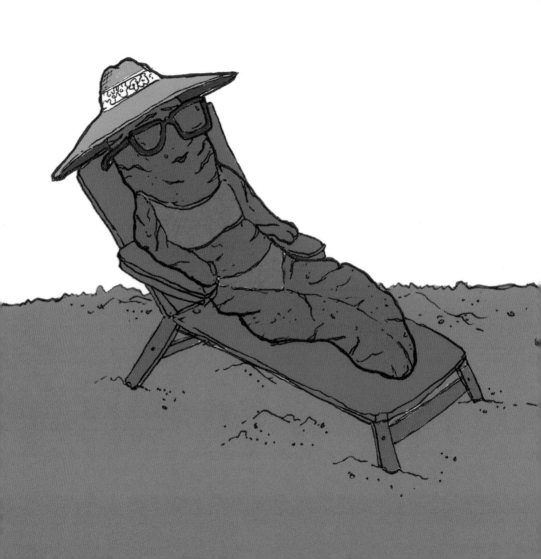

Half Baked

All dried up but this poop
has got a nice body.
Give her some water,
she'll dive right in the potty.

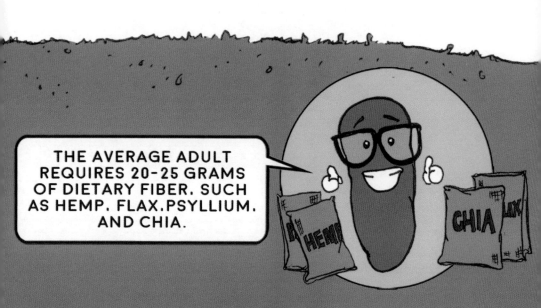

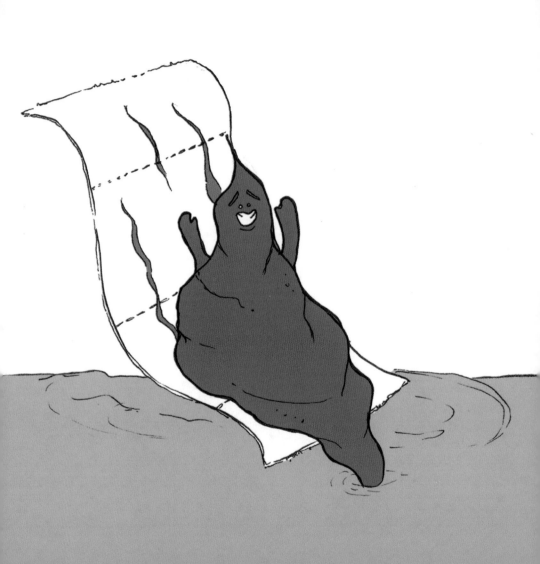

Stick-n-Slide

Sticky and wet
   he's sure to leave a mark.
Add in some fiber
   and wipe away the art.

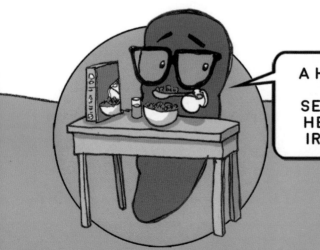

The Avalanche

Exploding from within,
  this avalanche erupts.
Sending debris flying
  straight out of your butt.

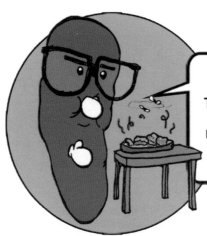

DIARRHEA CAN OCCUR
FROM EATING FOODS
THAT YOU ARE SENSITIVE
OR INTOLERANT TO.
USE OF LAXATIVES. MILD
FOOD POISONING. OR A
GUT INFECTION.

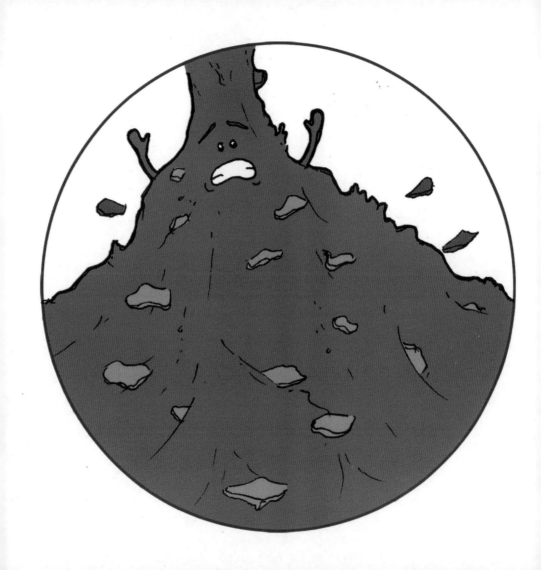

The Rafter

While water rafting
  on a dangerous rapid.
This watery mess
  needs electrolytes, fiber, and salad.

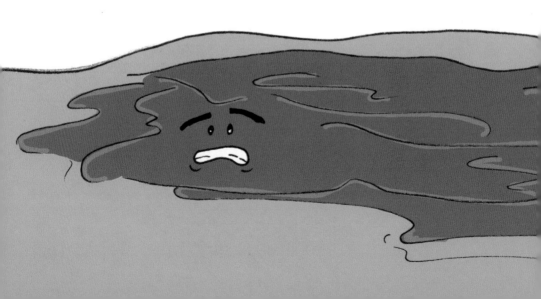

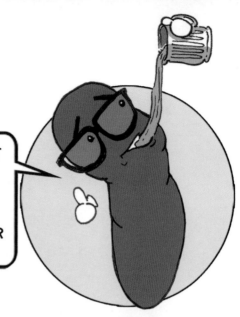
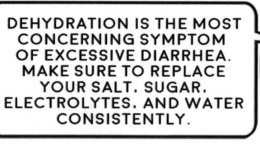

Greasy Floater

This greasy poop
   won't flush without a fight.
Fat malabsorption
   has him floating all night.

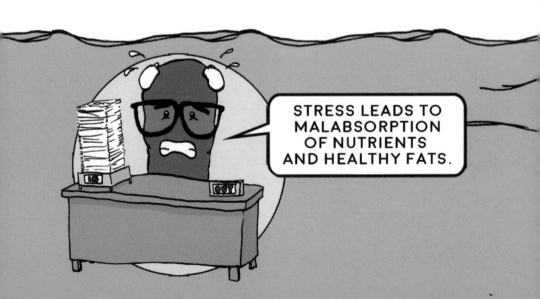

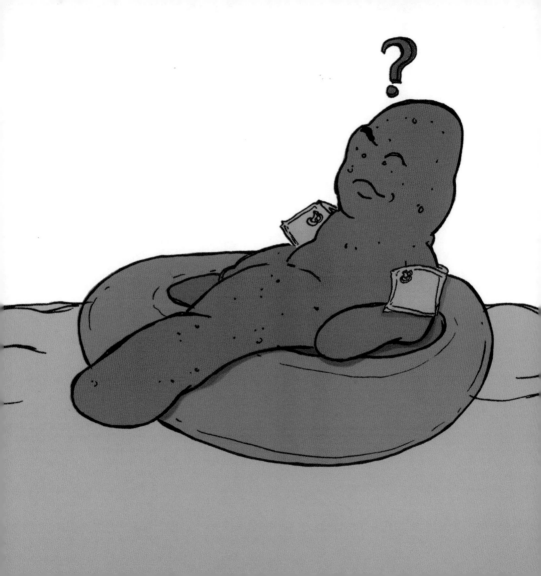

Chunky Stool

Undigested food
  can show up in your poo.
Don't eat in a hurry,
  chew through and through.

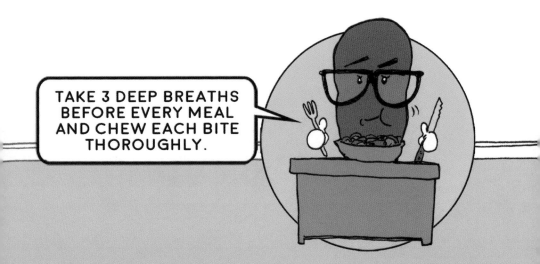

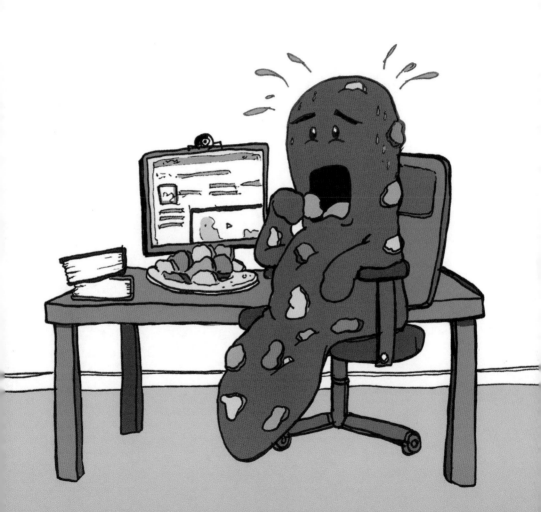

Itchy Bum

White little eggs
   and a very itchy bum,
Are signs that you have
   a parasite infection.

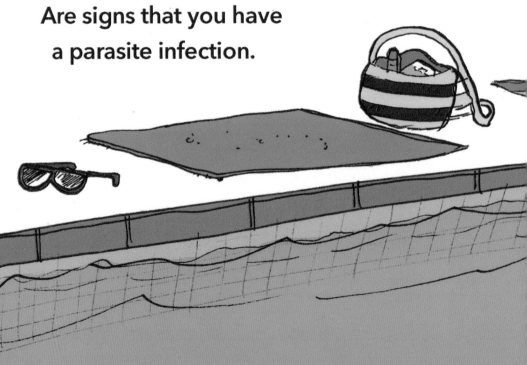

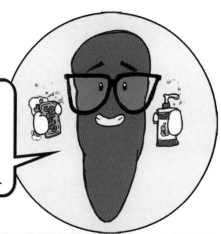

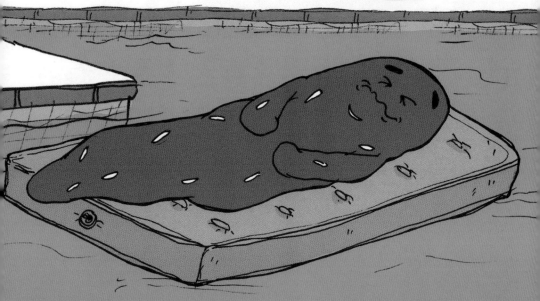

Stinky Butt

For all your issues

   with stinky poops, farts, and butts,

Balance your flora,

   eat greens, fruits, and nuts.

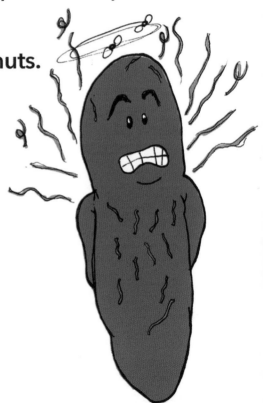

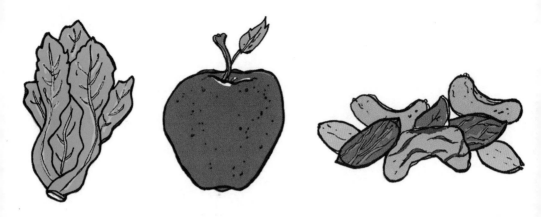

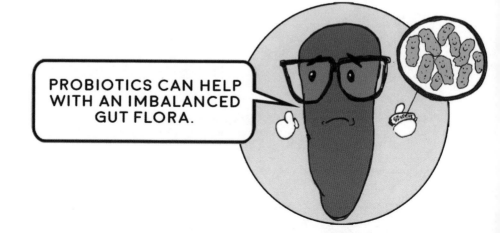

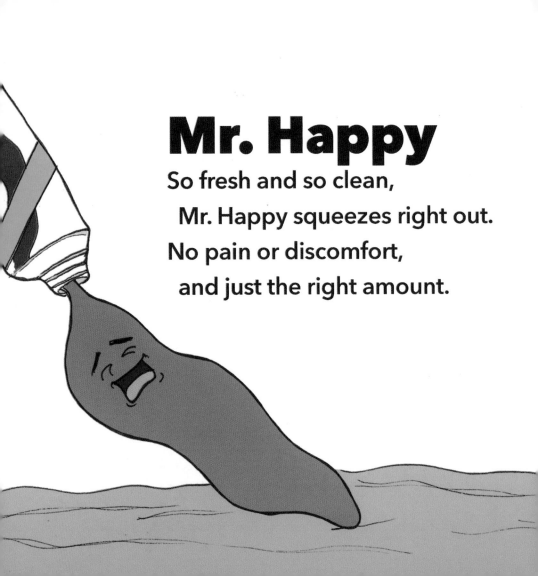

Mr. Happy

So fresh and so clean,
   Mr. Happy squeezes right out.
No pain or discomfort,
   and just the right amount.

A healthy brown color
is what we aspire,
Eating fiber and greens,
while drinking plenty of water.

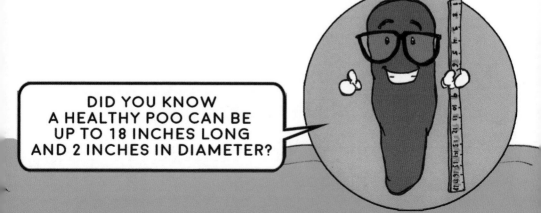

DID YOU KNOW
A HEALTHY POO CAN BE
UP TO 18 INCHES LONG
AND 2 INCHES IN DIAMETER?

Stools of the Rainbow

Bright red may represent
  a very dangerous color,
That indicates bleeding,
  a hemorrhoid or fissure.

Red can also be caused
  by the foods that you eat.
Have you recently had
  a red candy or red beet?

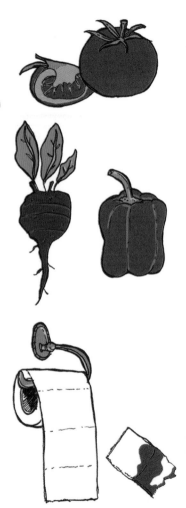

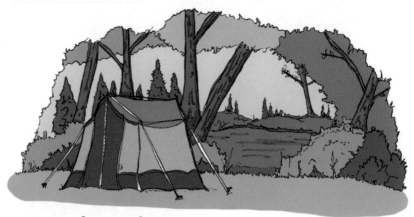

Green is the color
  of undigested bile,
Of antibiotics
  or eating leafy greens by the mile.

If your poop looks a bit yellow,
  get your gallbladder checked by a team.
But it might be a parasite
  from contaminated pork or a stream.

White or grey might be seen
  indicating blocked bile flow,
Disorders of the pancreas,
  or too many antacids in a row.

Danger is near
  with black, coffee ground poop,
A bleed might be high up
  in the intestinal loop.

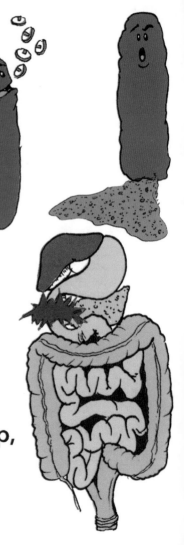

If you're doubled over in pain
and you ask yourself "why?",
Get a second opinion
to fix up your diet and GI.

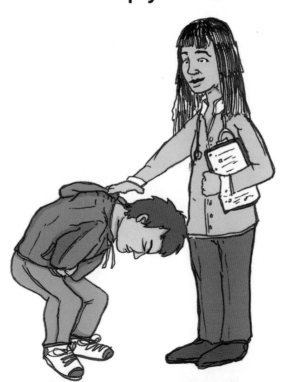
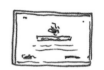
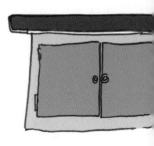

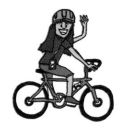 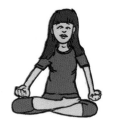 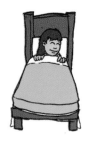

Exercise, meditation,
sunshine and rest,
Are other necessary factors
to poo without stress.

And remember to eat
all your greens, veggies and fruit,
And drink lots of water
for a healthier poop.

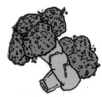 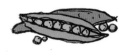 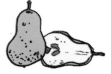

WHAT YOUR POO SAYS ABOUT YOU
COPYRIGHT © 2015 BY DR. ALISON CHEN. ND

ISBN-13: 978-1533590145
ISBN-10: 1533590141

BULK ORDER DISCOUNTS ARE AVAILABLE.
PLEASE EMAIL INFO@DRALISONCHEN.COM FOR ALL INQUIRIES.

PRINTABLE COLORING PAGES ARE FREE TO DOWNLOAD AT
WWW.DRALISONCHEN.COM/COLORME

ILLUSTRATIONS BY: JEREMY WAT

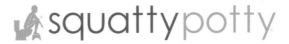

squattypotty

There's a Squatty for Everybody!

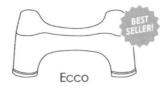

BEST SELLER!

Ecco

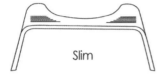

Slim

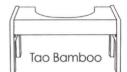

Tao Bamboo

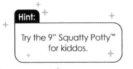

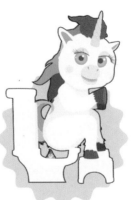

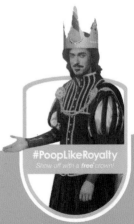

#PoopLikeRoyalty
Show off with a *free* crown!

Call toll-free
1.855.628.1099

Visit
squattypotty.com

*Exclusive to orders placed on squattypotty.com

Made in the USA
Lexington, KY
16 December 2016